Reduced to Madness

One Girl's Story About Surviving a Brain
Tumor and Postoperative PTSD

EXTENDED VERSION

BY
LAWANDA M BEYER

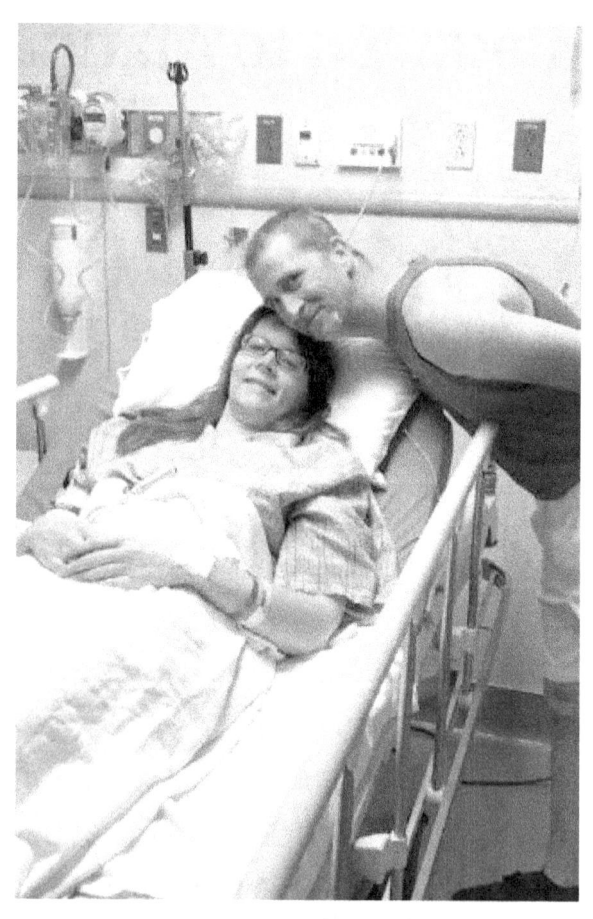

August 18, 2017

DEDICATION:

This book is dedicated to many.

My husband, Curt, who gently, graciously, and selflessly took care of me after my surgery and has taken care of me through everything that life has thrown at us. I will always be grateful to have you as my best friend, protector, and companion as we make our way through the madness. I love you.

My children, Joshua, and Hailey, for helping care for me through my hardest of times. Your mere existence and love is the sunshine in my life and has kept me fighting each day.

My parents, Merlin, and Callie, who crossed states and emotional turmoil to be by my side and help me recover.

My Aunt and prayer warrior, JoAnn, along with all my family & friends, churches, and even strangers who prayed on my behalf for a safe surgery and healing.

And foremost, to God, for showing me the true meaning of being grateful and the value of life in all things. And for giving me a deeper understanding of compassion, perseverance, and humility that I will carry with me for the rest of my days.

AUTHOR'S NOTES

Although they are all absolutely wonderful, I have left the identities of all my doctors, surgeons, and nurses out of this book for their own privacy.

My emotional turmoil has nothing to do with the amazing and tedious work they performed during my surgery and I am grateful I had such an amazing team. They did a wonderful job and saved my life. And I will be forever grateful to them all.

INTRODUCTION

I think back to the days when I was just a little girl. Playing in the sprinkler and laughing with my friends. Not a care in the world except for having fun and getting a popsicle while we dried in the sun. Then there were the teenage years. Then it was all about boys, the perfect figure, and what was in style. Girl secrets, skipping school, and prom. Sure, there were break ups and broken hearts and other things that I thought were the end of the world, but it was just the beginning of learning that life was not all about lollipops and rainbows.

Then, eventually I grew up. I fell madly in love and got married to the man I'm with today. We had our partying and we each had our own stupid mistakes but then babies started coming and life got real. We grew up. We started wearing our seat belts and stayed home on weekends. We got our first credit cards and loans and bought a house, a minivan, and a bunch of things we didn't need. We learned about responsibility real fast when debt and bills started stressing us out. It was life and we were living it. And of course we had our ups and downs and almost got divorced. Twice. Luckily, that's when we grew up some more and learned the real meaning of love and learned to be selfless and forgiving. And here we are today, still together and we've made it through it all.

I'm thinking back to all these things, my life memories... Me, the girl in the sprinkler. I remember her as I sit here now, at 41 years of age, still recovering from a brain surgery of ten months ago. Wow, the things that I worried about then. They all seem so petty compared to my recent wake up call. On August 18, I underwent an over 12 hour surgery to remove a large tumor that was pressing on my brain stem. It was the most horrible thing I have ever experienced and I am still recovering. At least I hope I am. I felt like I lost myself on that day. Unknowingly then, August 18th was the end of me as I knew myself, and the beginning of a different person. I am still me, but I am not. It's hard to explain, but in this book I will try.

I felt like someone threw me in the ocean on that day and I had been treading water ever since. And even though all my loved ones tried to help me through, it got more and more tiresome each day, like they were a million miles away. Even though they were right in front of me. And if I didn't find something to grab onto soon, I was going to drown.

Here is my story on surviving a brain tumor removal. The hell and recovery of it, and the postoperative PTSD that almost made me go insane.

---

in·sane / in ˈsān ; adjective
1. In a state of mind that prevents normal perception, behavior, or social interaction; seriously mentally ill.

CHAPTER ONE
THE DENIAL

"Mom, ... Mom, ... Hello, M-o-t-h-e-r?"

This is where it all began to hit me. I was literally losing my hearing. My daughter was trying to speak to me and I didn't hear a word she said until she stood straight in front of my face with a worried and questioning look. I knew my ears had been plugged and my hearing had slowly faded a bit, but I didn't realize the severity until this day. I snapped my fingers in front of my left ear, and nothing.

Backing up a bit, I had always had issues with my ears due to a condition called TMJ. Temporomandibular joint disorder. TMJ is a condition of the temporomandibular joint, which is a hinge connecting your jaw to the part of your skull in front of your ears. I obtained this condition after a four hour wisdom tooth removal by a quack dentist. My jaw was open for all four hours, aching, and stressed. Also, my teeth roots were wrapped around my jawbone. I should have been taken to an oral surgeon, but unfortunately, at that time in my life, I was broke and had no dental insurance. I opted for the cheapest dental place I could find, which was out of his house mind you, red flag, but I was like 19 and had no good sense. He had to

remove my wisdom teeth each in eight pieces and also remove part of my jaw bone. Anyway, the dentist accomplished the task and I didn't die, and my mouth healed. But unfortunately I was left with TMJ. Something I now look back on and laugh at. Because of everything I had ever gone through in my life, TMJ was piddle compared to what was coming.

So, moving on, often my TMJ would cause me headaches, off bite, and a plugged feeling in my ears. You can see how my condition would not alarm me of having any other new issues other than my normal TMJ. I lived with TMJ for many years until one fortunate day, I met a wonderful Chiropractor in our nearby town of Ardmore, Oklahoma. Dr. Lee Grant. After listening to my complaints, he adjusted my jaw and literally in about 5 seconds my TMJ symptoms were gone. It was like a miracle! My bite was right on, my ears unplugged, and I felt great!

But, gradually my ears would still plug up and I blamed it on needing to hit the chiropractor's office again. Little did I know or realize, that my plugging ears were also the sign of a deeper issue within my head. One that had been slowly developing for a long time.

After my daughter made me realize just how bad my hearing had gotten, I admit I did procrastinate going to a doctor. It scared me a little bit and I tried to just not think about it, I thought I was going to have to have TMJ surgery and that would suck. I always heard nightmares about people having to get their jaw wired shut, and nope, that was just not happening to me. But after many nudges from my worried husband asking me to go get my ears checked out, and a nudge from my chiropractor, Dr. Grant, I finally made an appointment with our local ENT to have a hearing test done.

The appointment for my hearing test was weeks out, so life went on as normal. I went to work and went about my daily routines. I did however, start to notice that my balance was off. I stumbled into things once in a while and would feel a little odd at times but I blamed that on being over tired. I also had tinnitus in my bad ear. Just a very quiet humming, like the sound of a florescent light in a quiet library. But I quickly tossed everything to just being clumsy and over tired. I worked seven days a week doing demanding, stressful paperwork and reports. I never gave anything a serious or second thought.

Then one day, my husband and I went to a furniture store to look at some bedroom sets. This store was in an old downtown building with two stories. It had a very long and wide staircase to get to the second floor. Going up was no big deal. We looked around at a lot of stuff and then when it came time to go back down to the main floor, I looked at the stairs before me and dizziness and anxiety hit me. I felt like I was going to fall and break my neck if I didn't grab my husband's arm. It was almost as if the room started to rotate. So I held onto him and started down the stairs. I kind of joked about my fear of heights and that was my last thought about it and the day went on.

APPOINTMENT DAY

"Nothing is really real...
until it slaps you in the face."

My ENT appointment day had finally arrived. I was at work on a normal day, plucking away at my paperwork, waiting for my appointment to come around. My husband and I both work at the same office for an oilfield company. Our desks are right across from each other. He normally is out doing shop or field work, so he wasn't there when I left for my appointment. I headed out alone to go get the hearing test done. No big deal. I knew they were just going to say I had TMJ and everything I already knew. Worse case scenario, I was getting old and

needed a hearing aid, HAHA, a little joke in my head. All I was really thinking about was my husband's birthday coming up. It was on May 22nd, and I was still trying to think of some grand birthday surprise.

Anyway, I left work that day and I arrived at my appointment. I checked in and sat in the waiting room as to be expected. They eventually called me back to a room where hearing tests are done. There was this little padded booth with a chair, some headphones, and other gadgets. I got the headphones put on and they went through their routine of having me listen to words and repeat what I heard. This was done for both ears separately and together. My right ear was great. I wasn't too nervous as I felt I was hearing everything pretty good. Then my left. It was weak but I could hear a little. All was good. That is, until the audiologist told me that what I was hearing was coming from my right ear, not my left. Supposedly my right ear was picking up some slack. So then he plugged my right ear with some distracting noise and tested only the left. And I could barely hear a thing.

I remember getting a little nervous as it seemed the audiologist was writing a novel on my paperwork. He had me exit the hearing booth and sit on a chair.

He told me I had hearing loss in my left ear and a condition causing me to be unable to tell which direction sound was coming from. A light bulb went off in my head as I thought to myself and realized that I run in the opposite direction to find my ringing cell phone all the time. Then he sent me to wait in another room to talk to the doctor. I remember clearly getting a glimpse of his chart as I stood up and seeing the words "SEVERE" in big red marker on his paperwork. I was thinking in my head that it was a little odd and alarming for him to have made a big note like that. But I proceeded to the other exam room and awaited the doctor to come in.

When the doctor entered the room, she smiled, shook my hand, and looked at my paperwork as she started asking me questions like, have you had any tinnitus? Have you been losing your balance? Did your hearing loss come on suddenly or gradually? Etc. I reassured her that it was gradually and that I have TMJ, so it was normal to feel plugged up in the head and so on. But she just smiled, nodded, and proceeded to tell me that I needed to have an MRI of my brain, as it was not normal to have this severity of hearing loss at my age. And she assured me that TMJ was not the cause. She then proceeded to apologize to me like someone had just passed away, and told me she believed I had a brain tumor. Of course they couldn't be sure, but it was either that, or I had a viral infection that took my hearing. But, more likely, a brain tumor.

Wait. What?

There was a moment of silence and denial in my head. I kind of tuned her out at that moment as she explained how they would set everything up. All I could think about was that I was going to die. I wouldn't see my kids get married, I wouldn't see my grandchildren, and life just hit me with a bitch slap that stung like hell.

Wait, her mouth was moving, but I have no idea what she all just said. I was dreaming. Wake me up!

She apologized to me like my days were numbered and she left the room.

I don't even really remember what happened after all that other than all of a sudden I was sitting in my car in the parking lot and I could not start the car. My heart started pounding, I couldn't breath, and the world was closing in on me. I sat there for about an hour crying my eyes out and thinking the worst. My chest felt like it was going to explode with emotion.

Should I call my husband? Should I call my parents? Should I go home? Should I go back to work? Should I start a will? I couldn't even think straight. I was numb and yet I felt every emotion all at once. It didn't feel real that this was really happening. To me. I'm just LaWanda. This bomb is not allowed to fall on me! What did I do to deserve this? Oh my God, my kids... my kids. I can't leave my kids.

I finally calmed down enough to wipe my face and start the car. I took a long deep breath. And I gave myself an imaginary slap in the face and decided it was going to be no big deal. It was probably just a virus or some misunderstanding. What do doctors know anyway?! I'll just keep it to myself until I have the MRI and get some results. End of discussion.

CHAPTER 2
MY BALANCING ROD

I drove back to work as planned for that day and planned to go on as if nothing had changed. But as soon as I got into the office and sat at my desk, my husband came in. And seeing him, and thinking about how much I loved him, immediately I produced the waterworks all over again!

Knowing that I had just come from my ear appointment, he had the most shocked and concerned look on his face. I could barely mutter the words of the results of my appointment to him as I gasped for air from sobbing so deeply. For a moment he was frozen. I could see the traumatized fear in his face after the words "brain tumor" finally came from my mouth.

Time stood still for a moment, but then he hugged me and quickly assured me that everything would be fine. He said we shouldn't think the worst when we hadn't even had the MRI yet. I shook my head in agreeance as he wiped my face. I knew he flipped his emotional coin for my benefit. I could tell he pushed his own fears aside to calm and protect my mind and keep me positive. And I loved him for that. He was my rock, my balance rod, and focal point. He kept me together. When he was by my side I was grounded and safe.

I had never been so grateful to have this man. When I would start to get down and let fear take over, he was there in my face, wiping my tears, and looking me in the eyes, and bringing me back to center. I couldn't imagine anyone having to go through this alone. It was terrifying and life changing. If it weren't for my husband, my mind and life would have spiraled out of control at this point.

MRI DAY

It seemed to take forever for the MRI appointment day to arrive. In waiting, each day I had some sort of crying spell in thinking the worst. I wanted to be strong, but inside I was as scared as a lost child in a mega mall. But each time my mind started going to bad places, I shook it off. I put on my big girl attitude, and went on with my day. My husband's words of "we got this" played over and over in my head.

When the day finally came, I remember how cold and nervous I was. They put an IV in my arm for the dye and submitted my body into the giant space chamber. Being a supernatural and science fiction fan, in my mind, I pretended I was somewhere else to ease the nervousness. The machine made all it's swirling and banging noises as my mind drifted off to a place of disbelief and imagination. Of course everything was going to come out fine. There would be no tumor. I was just a regular haphazard girl who was going to end up with a huge bill to pay.

After the MRI was over, I collected a disc to drop off to my ENT doctor for review. Of course I popped that puppy in my laptop to spy on the contents before swinging by the ENT. After all, I wasn't going to wait forever for this kind of news. So, my husband figured out how to get the files open and we skimmed through the images. At first it just looked like normal brainy stuff, we flipped through the thousands of images. I was just starting to think, Ha! Pffhah! Nothing! And then there it was. A large white mass that didn't look like it belonged. We weren't brain experts, but it was pretty obvious that I had an uninvited object in my head. My husband played it off as if we still didn't have definite answers, but I knew that my life was about to change, and all of a sudden everything got very real. And very scary.

I dropped the disc off to the ENT and we had to wait a little while for the doctor to get back to us on the results. And needless to say, my mind was playdough. I felt like I was in a daze most of the time, wishing someone would just pinch me and I would wake up. But there was no pinch and there was no waking up from this dream.

My ENT doctor eventually contacted me confirming that I indeed had a brain tumor called an acoustic neuroma, also known as a Vestibular Schwannoma. She assured me these were usually non-cancerous types of tumors, although mine was very large and pressing on my brain stem. She advised it be taken care of as soon as possible. Her office set me up with an appointment at a place that removed tumors, but my mind was not at ease. I felt like I needed to do some digging on more professionals available. After all, this was my brain we were talking about, and I didn't want just anyone digging around in my head. So we started doing our digging on the internet and looking for the best doctors for the job.

Eventually we agreed on a place is Dallas that dealt specifically with the brain and tumors, and they had impeccable reviews. I knew in my heart that it was where I needed to go for my operation. I called my ENT back and asked that they refer me to this place and they agreed. They faxed over my information to them on May 24th. The Dallas specialists called me back the same day with an appointment for June 13th. This would be a consult appointment with some testing. So three weeks of

waiting and thinking. I could do this. Right? Well, three weeks to think and fidget felt like three months. And meanwhile, my balance was getting worse and I felt like I was spiralling quickly.

It was kind of ironic that I later found out that May was brain tumor month. A month that suddenly would become an emotional pin on my brain's memory cork board. At first I was feeling kind of

cursed. But I knew cursed was not in my news feed because once word was out about my condition, I had never ending love and overwhelming support from my family and friends. Churches, prayer chains, and personal pleas were going up for my peace, safe operation, and complete recovery. I had friends in China, Russia, Ukraine, and in the U.S., I had people from all walks of the earth praying, chanting, and burning sweet grasses. Divine intervention in every form was being beckoned for my sake. And it strengthened me, gave me hope, and most of all, it gave me faith. I truly believed that whatever happened, and whatever I would go through, in the end, it was all going to be okay. God was on my side, and I needed to stay focused on that.

CHAPTER 3
OFF TO DALLAS

The day finally came when we headed out the door to go to Dallas and talk to the brain specialists. We went over the MRI and what options we had and which ones were best for my case. They confirmed that I had a large tumor called an acoustic neuroma, also known as, a vestibular schwannoma. They said I was past having the option of any radiation as it was a very large tumor and it was pressing on my brain stem and facial nerves. Not removing it would eventually cause major nerve damage and eventually death. They were very upfront with me in saying that the surgery would be very long, over 10 hours, and difficult to perform. They said it could result in some facial nerve damage along with other possible difficulties.

All these things made me very nervous. But at this point I had no choice. Take it out and chance facial paralysis and other issues, or eventually let this foreign object kill me. So we proceeded with the plan of having it removed.

I had to return to Dallas again before surgery to see the ear surgeon who would be performing the ear part of the surgery.

They explained that the safest way to get in to remove the tumor would be through the ear and around the outside of the brain as much as possible and to the back of my head, near my brain stem. They would be removing my entire inner ear and I would be left completely deaf on my left side.

Deaf in one ear... this was disturbing to me, but still, I would be alive. And I had already lost most of my hearing anyway, so I was keeping my chin up.

I returned to see the ear surgeon and have some balance and nerve testing done. All the tests they put my ears and brain through made me very sick. I rode home, a two hour trip, with my head in my husband's lap as the world spun and I felt like I was going to vomit. As soon as we got home, I went straight to bed with what felt like a terrible case of the tummy bug and extreme dizziness. The Dr. said that seeing how badly I took the testing, the surgery was going to make me very ill. Most likely for days. So I dreaded feeling that again. But I tried to stay positive. A few days of feeling sick, then I 'll be back to myself and have my head back. Right?

My surgery was scheduled for July 21st. About a week out. But then the next day I got a call that they were adding a third surgeon and there was a conflict in their schedules, so my surgery was moved to August 18th. I was upset, I just wanted this to be over, but at the same time, I was kind of happy that I had some time to just be me. Just in case something went wrong. No, nothing is going to go wrong. I needed to stop that negative thinking. God is just moving things around for his perfect timing. Yes, that's better. God is in control.

Every day that went by before my surgery, I tried to stay calm and put on a strong front. I tried my hardest to stay positive and have faith. I meditated, I prayed, and I just listened to nature. I tried to take in the little things and appreciate my family. I guess you could say that I was just doing some emotional prep, maybe some soul searching. I would find myself just laying on my bed, closing my eyes, and thinking about all the little memories of my life. My kids being born, what wind felt like on my face, just all kinds of thoughts. No rhyme or reason.

CHAPTER 4
THE ZEBRA

One afternoon, I was lying on my bed. My eyes were closed. I was just taking in my breath but I was wide awake. And in the darkness of my eyelids a zebra walked upon me. Like a vision. It came so close to me that I could see all the details of its eye. I don't know what that was all about but it seemed significant. The zebra's eye was so clear and beautiful. My heart palpitated just a little bit as I experienced this vision with such clarity. When I opened my eyes, I knew that this had to be some sort of sign. It seemed odd that of all things, I saw a zebra, or anything at all, but it felt significant. And I felt like God had just visited with me and I felt peaceful yet a little scared. What did it mean?

I asked my Aunt, who has experience in visions and the sort, what she thought about my zebra experience. I also looked up zebra symbols on the internet. Some things that stood out to me were that supposedly the zebra stood for turning negative life experiences into positive ones, or vice versa. Basically that a change was coming, and you can find a balance in it, or see it differently all together. But it stressed a significant change was coming and that new knowledge could be obtained.

This really struck me straight in the heart. I was getting ready to have brain surgery. I knew my life was about to change, and I also knew that no matter what happened in the outcome, I would learn something from the experience. Good or bad, I was about to go down an unknown path. And I could either make the best of it, or just be miserable, but I decided to make the best of it. I tried to keep faith in what I believed, and that was that God was with me. And everything would be okay.

EMOTIONAL ROLLER COASTER

I'm going to be honest. After everything I just said about the zebra and being positive, well... much easier said than done. As surgery day got closer and closer, I started to feel like I was in a love/hate relationship with my feelings and my faith. I would be positive one day and crying the next. Praising God one day, and doubting him the next. And I feel ashamed to admit that, but I was just an emotional mess, and most of it was kept neatly and quietly in my mind. I didn't want to burden my overworked husband or worry my distant family, so I just dealt with all my feelings alone. I would cry in my car and smile at work. I was alone inside myself, wearing a warriors pose. And I shouldn't have done that to myself.

CHAPTER 5
SURGERY ARRIVES

The day before my surgery, I was surprisingly not as nervous as I thought I would be. I knew I had the prayers of many churches, all of my friends, coworkers, family, and even people I didn't even know. And the support I received from everyone was amazing. It made me feel at peace. Even though, I still had that tiny knot in my gutt. After all, I was about to go get my head cut open, I also knew I had chosen the best surgeons around to care for me. I felt as if God was truly in my corner at this moment. Like He was holding his umbrella over my head. And I tried to stand strong on the feeling.

We all decided as a family that it was best that our two teens stayed home. It was going to be a long surgery, at least ten hours, and they wouldn't see me for at least two days afterwards because I would be in ICU. I didn't want them pacing the hospital with anxieties and fears. Or sitting in a hotel room alone just waiting. I also didn't want them to see me all miserable. So I assured them everything would be fine and they should stay home and do their normal routines. Watch movies, talk with their friends, and play with our dogs. And they were content with that and the fact that Dad would keep them updated.

It was hard to say goodbye to the kids when we left that night, but it put my mind at ease that they had each other to keep company. And being a mom, It feared me to think that if they came with, they would be driving about the big city when I was having surgery. So I was glad that they were staying home. Kind of funny, right? I was about to have brain surgery, but I was mostly worried about my children. Anyway, it was decided. They were staying home safe and sound, and that was that.

My parents were also planning a 13 hour drive from Minnesota to come be with me in the hospital, but like the kids, I told them to wait until I got home. They would only have a week or two to be with us because of my dad's work and I didn't want their time wasted on not being able to see me for a few days. I rathered they be with me during my recovery. So they planned to head down as soon as they heard I was going home. And I felt badly for them having to wait, because I can only imagine how I would feel if it were my child in the hospital. And I knew my mother was probably having enough anxiety to lift a small building. But we all eventually agreed it best to wait for them to come until I was comfortably home. Then they could spend all their time with me and help out as needed.

My surgery was scheduled for early morning and we had a two hour drive into Texas to get to the hospital, so we made the trip the night before and stayed in a hotel that our friend, and boss, Jerrod, who owned the oilfield company we both worked for, had ever so generously reserved for us for a whole week so that my husband could be comfortable. Jerrod also booked a room at the hotel for himself and accompanied us to eating dinner and catching a movie that night. It was pleasant and helpful in keeping my mind off of what was about to happen in the morning. Needless to say, my husband and I were very grateful to have such a supportive boss and friend.

Although they all wanted to be there, all of our family was out of state except for my sister, and they had a virus keeping them home, and my husband had nobody to be with him at the hospital. So it really eased my mind knowing that Jerrod was going to be with him while I was in surgery for so long. I didn't want him pacing alone for 10 hours thinking the worst. I will never forget, and always appreciate, everything Jerrod had done for us.

When we returned to our hotel for the evening, I got ready for bed, packed my hospital bag, and tried to go to sleep. I called my parents and left messages on their phones just to say that I loved them. Just in case. Then, I laid awake in bed for quite some time. I won't forget the constant buzzing noise that came

from outside our window, and the thoughts that were going through my mind. Negative thoughts of not making it through the surgery and never seeing my family again haunted me for a short while. I was worried that I would wake up from surgery paralyzed, or not at all. It was hard to fall asleep, but I said a prayer and eventually I managed to drift off.

Surgery Day

It felt like two seconds had gone by when our alarm went off that morning. I was so tired and my husband kind of joked that I could go back to sleep soon. You know, for 10 hours. I remember trying not to think about anything. Just get ready for the day, get to the hospital, and do this thing. I told myself I got this and I just want to get it over with. I'm going to wake up from surgery, everything will be awesome, I won't be paralyzed, my face will still work, I will feel like a million bucks riding on a unicorn. Okay? Good.

I must have gone into a small sleepwalking fear coma, because the next thing I remember at this point was being in the prep room. I remember laying in the hospital bed with those rolling curtains surrounding my bed. My husband, boss, and anesthesiologist standing there with all their best wishes of how everything would be fine.

Now, let me step back a few days for a moment to explain something that transpired at my pre-surgery doctor appointment. The doctor had asked me who would be there for me on surgery day. And she asked me something about having more than one spouse. My husband and I laughed and I replied that only my husband would be there. And then the doctor explained to us that she had to ask this because some people did in fact surprise the staff by awkwardly bringing in more than one spouse, or a secret lover. We laughed, it was interesting, and then I assured them only my husband would be with me. Mind you, that was before I knew that Jerrod was coming along.

Now back to surgery prep... I remember the surgeon popping in for a moment to ease my mind and nonchalantly ask who the other gentleman was with me. My husband and I laughed as we both realized what he was probably thinking. But, we assured him, that the gentlemen was our friend, and boss, no surprise lovers here, lol. The doctor chuckled and mentioned how lucky we were to have such a supportive boss.

I had to laugh inside because I wondered if other staff thought I had two lovers with me, hahaha! Anyway, it was kind of funny. The whole thing kind of lifted some anxiety for a moment and I felt in good spirits.

A little comical story I would remember on a crazy scarey day.

Then, my mind started drifting. The anesthesiologist's mouth was moving but all I could hear were my own thoughts of how I got this, everything will be ok, it's almost over, what if I die, my parents must be going crazy by now, ok, stay calm, my kids ....ZZzzzzZZZZZZzzzzzzzzzz....
and I was out for the count.

CHAPTER 6
TO HELL AND BACK

*"LaWanda, can you hear me? It's your Dr., LaWanda?...
LaWanda are you with us?"*

After my surgery, which ended up taking 12 hours, I
woke up to voices that faded in from a dream that I
don't remember. Everything was bright, cold, loud,
and then **BARF**. The surgeon's flashlight was
blinding me, everything was blurry, and I started
vomiting non-stop. What little bit of puke I had in
my stomach was just running down my chin. I
couldn't move my face. I could feel the empty pit in
my stomach and the burning of the vomit on my
face. The nurses were wiping the vomit from my
numb chin and rubbing my back. My head felt like it
weighed 80 pounds and the room was spinning so
fast that I had to grip my sheets and keep my eyes
closed. All I could do was vomit, dry heave, and
hold onto the bed. It felt like I was going to fly off of
it like the exorcist. The spinning and nausea were
so intense and never ending that I actually wished
death upon myself. I just wanted to ease my own
suffering.

The first couple of days I could not get out of bed or
eat anything. I would try to sip water but it just ran

down my face. I eventually learned to use a straw in a way that would assist me to drink.

The surgeon said they had to peel my facial nerve off of my brain stem and that my facial nerve was traumatized because of it. But they had high hopes that my facial paralysis would end and that I would return to normal in maybe a year.

I had a lot of adjusting to do after my surgery. My head was sawed open, a tumor removed, fat from my abdomen was taken and put in my head, along with a titanium mesh plate. My left inner ear was removed during surgery. It left me deaf in one ear. The world around me sounded different. Everything sounded like it was underwater and muffled. My face didn't work, and my eyes were very dry. My tear duct in my left eye quit working. I had to put artificial tears in every hour or my eye felt like sandpaper. And my entire head had ringing that was so loud I could barely stand it. You can compare it to when you are watching a movie and a bomb goes off near people and they are disoriented and left with piercing ringing. That is how I felt. I felt carried out of battle wounded. My husband played music to try to ease my irritation, of which that actually did help. I also lost my taste buds and everything tasted like butter.

Every night in the hospital I had tormenting nightmares. Not nightmares like a person would normally have, but more like repetitive images that I could not wake up from. I remember one night I was stuck in my own mind. All I could see was the inside of my skull and it was full of bloody branches, or maybe veins, that were growing and entangling each other. Smothering and strangling my brain to death. My heart was pounding, I was terrified, and I could not wake up. I remember wanting to wake up so bad that I was screaming inside of myself. Finally a nurse woke me out of my sleep to give me an anxiety pill. She said my heart rate was sky high. I was so grateful that she woke me up because I felt like I was going to die.

Another night I was again, stuck inside my skull, but this time it was with all kinds of patterns that twisted and turned. I felt like I was in a maze of dizziness that I could not escape from. It is very hard to describe, and it may not sound scary, but it was unbelievably traumatic. I felt like my brain was having nightmares, not me. My brain was stuck in groundhogs day, nightmare edition. Sometimes I wonder if my brain was having nightmares from not being able to wake up. Like it was held down by 12 hours of anesthesia, kept prisoner and unable to communicate with my body. It felt like my brain was screaming for help and confused.

Between the nightmares, lack of sleep, loud ringing, extreme dizziness, and nausea, I didn't want another day to pass. And I most certainly was not expecting the recovery I was handed. God where are you?...

A few days after my surgery, I was finally forced to sit up. It was hard to sit without falling over. But each day did bring it's tiny improvement until I finally had a walker and was able to walk little bits at a time. The world still spinning, I felt like I fought gravity everyday just to take a step and stay upright. I worried everyday that my balance would never come back. But my husband did his best to keep me positive and pushed me to what I was able. I held his arm tightly as I forced myself to walk through the hospital halls. Halls that felt like a spinning funhouse, except nobody was having any fun.

The day came when I finally made a lap around the nurse's station. I remember how proud my husband was. He had been holding onto me, inching me further each day, and when I made it all the way around, it was like he just saw his 1 year old walk for the first time. It was an emotional day. He was proud, I was encouraged a little bit, but still facing the fight of each day.

And every night the nightmares returned, my ears rang, the room spun, and as if things were not bad enough, yup, I got my period. And that for me is a misery in itself, as I have endometriosis and have very heavy and painful periods. So there was that to deal with as well.

With my husband's assistance, I finally managed to get a shower, my long hair was such a rats nest that my poor husband could not comb it out. Bless the nurse that came in and carefully combed out all of my snarls. Working her way around the stitches and staples that lined the side of my head, she put a braid in my hair. And I will never forget that.

The surgeons visited me on a couple occasions to check on me and observe my balance and nerves. They said my outlook was good. They believed I would get most of my facial movement back and that my balance would improve over time. They explained that I had the deepest cranial surgery a person could have, and that it would take time to heal. And I could expect headaches, stabbing pains, and possibly depression. I was to eat a high protein diet, get some walking in, but to not over do it, as my body would use all its calories to heal my skull, so nap, rest, eat, and watch for spinal drainage.

And so I was soon released to the care of my husband and we got ready to go home with instruction to return in a few weeks for a follow-up

MRI. All together, I was in the hospital for a week. I lost 30 lbs and a part of myself.

CHAPTER 7
GOING HOME

I will never forget the day that I was released to go home. My husband and a nurse wheeled me down to the main floor. The nurse and I sat outside and waited for my husband to bring the truck around. It felt like I hadn't been outside in forever. I just sat in the wheelchair taking in all the fresh air. It was the perfect temperature outside with a slight breeze. I remember the sound and feeling of the mylar balloons gently hitting my shoulder. And the breeze blowing my hair. I just closed my eyes and took it all in.

My husband pulled up front and I was gently assisted into the truck along with my bags, plants and balloons that were sent to me. As we drove away from the hospital I felt a little nervous about going home and not having all those handy nurses, but I knew my parents were on their way soon and I was excited to see them. Riding in the truck for two hours to get home was a little nauseating. I felt like the world was still spinning. And I could hear everything. The sound of the truck, traffic, and construction. Everything seemed magnified and a little overwhelming. Any little bumps in the road made my head throb.

On our way home, I actually started to feel hungry. Pretty much all I had in the hospital were scrambled eggs, pediasure, and jello. The only thing in the world that sounded good now was chicken nuggets and a soda! So we hit a drive thru and ordered just that. Unfortunately, my taste buds were still on strike and the soda tasted awful. I couldn't even drink it. Oddly, the nuggets weren't that bad.

On arriving home, I was so happy to see my kids! They were so happy and gentle to hug me and get me comfortable in my chair. I felt horrible and dizzy, but tried to put on a good front for their sake. I could see the shock in their faces when they seen that my face was paralyzed. But they tried to act as if nothing was different. But, I knew they were a little surprised by my appearance.

It felt good to be home and surrounded by my family. It was nice to be done with the poking and prodding. But I think this is where my depression started to kick in. For the first time, I was able to be alone. I would have assistance to the bathroom or bedroom or wherever I needed to go, but then I had time alone to look at myself in the mirror. I looked at my face and it's drooping and it felt like I was looking at someone else. I felt like a stranger to myself and I felt ugly and incompetent. I couldn't do anything on my own. I had a shower seat to sit on and my husband washed me. He combed my hair, dressed me, helped me walk and stand. I never imagined that I would be learning to live all over again, but that was basically what I had to do. I had to learn to walk again, eat, drink, brush my teeth, spit, shower, and get dressed. I felt myself slowly going into a dark place of self pity and sadness. I was miserable, uncomfortable, and irritated.

I spent most of my time in my recliner napping, and just trying to stand being alive. The room spun, my head hurt, and I felt helpless. When my parents arrived, a wave of happiness finally came over me. I hadn't seen them in so long, and seeing and feeling their embrace was overwhelmingly emotional. My head throbbed and my chest hurt from the emotions that expanded inside of me. It felt so good to have them with me. I felt like a little girl who needed her mom again. And nothing was more soothing than feeling mom and dad's gentle hug and just smelling them and hearing them nearby. They were a great comfort and support to me starting to heal.

One day in particular is embedded forever in my memories. The day my dad helped me put on some shoes, took my hands, and led me outside without my walker. He held my hands the whole time and guided me on a short walk on the driveway. I felt like his little toddler learning to walk again. And he had me. He encouraged me to push myself just enough to start rehabilitating. As miserable as I felt, the doctors said I needed to be doing this. Sitting in my chair all day wouldn't help my brain heal or learn to balance itself. And after that, we took a little bit longer walks each day until I finally tried the treadmill. It was short, but it was something.

Although I was improving a tiny bit each day, it still felt like one step forward and two steps back. My ears started ringing worse and worse and it was maddening. Like holding a fire alarm right up to your ear and it not shutting off. I had to play music and noise makers in every room to try to distract myself. And my dry tear ducts were causing shooting pains in my eye which brought on headaches. But I had to keep pushing on each day. And every night my husband would prop up all my pillows, get me comfortable in bed, bring me a big glass of water, make sure I took my pills, and he would crawl in bed and encourage me with something positive to say. Then I would eventually drift off to a very welcoming sleep. An escape from the dizziness and misery of the day.

EVERY CRUEL DAY

I'm standing barefoot in the creek. The ice cold water is flowing over my feet. I watch the water as it passes through my wiggling toes. It's just a simple moment of peace in my head. I can almost feel the breeze as it gently wisps through my hair. Then, I wake up and the moment is gone. I wake up to my noise maker. It was just a dream. But for that moment I felt normal. Sleep was my only relief. When I was asleep in my bed, it was like nothing existed. I would count down the moments of the day until I could just sleep again. Sleeping was escaping. But, there I lay, awake now in my bed. It's morning and I am afraid to open my eyes. I know as soon as I acknowledge the day and open my eyes, the room will be spinning like a hell ride at the fair. And nobody gets off this ride all day. At least I don't. I tell myself over and over that I can make it through one more day. I try to sit up in bed and the spinning and unbalance has me ready spew vomit. I fumble for my eyeglasses and try to get out of bed. My husband has his hands out so I can reach for him and all I can think of is how I don't want to go through one more day feeling like this. But with his help, I make it to the bathroom and he helps me center on the toilet so I can go pee. All while holding on to him so I do not sway over and fall off of the toilet. All I can think about is how it's so humiliating, as I hold on to him and try to wipe and stand up so he can help me with my pajamas. Thank God all I had to do was pee. That thought went through my mind many times. He was gentle and willing, but the fact that I could not care for my basic needs was killing me.

My husband constantly assured me that I was going to make it through this. He was a refreshing constant reminder that the spinning would get better and I would get back to myself. Time, it just all takes time, he would say. I know, I know! But let me tell you that it is very hard to wait for time when you are miserable. It felt like I had a knife jabbed in my skull, my hair was falling out and in a tangled mess. It hurt to have it combed. But everyday, as the doctor ordered, I would fight the spinning and feel my way to the shower. I used a walker of course and had constant supervision. And when I say constant, I mean, my husband even had to get in the shower with me while I sat on a shower chair, and bless his heart, he bathed me, gently washed my hair around all my staples and stitches, and even shaved my legs. He dried me off, got me dressed, and helped me to stand at the sink so I could brush my teeth. Even brushing my teeth was a challenge with half my face paralysed. I would brush the best I could and try to rinse, but the water would just run out my mouth and down my chin. And so I had to clean up my face, cry, and try to stay positive. Acne was breaking out all over my face and it looked like my skin was just going to slide right off my face. But I tried to stay positive. Positive. Positive. I am going to get through this. No I'm not. Yes I am. Now here come the waterworks again, well, out of one eye anyway. So I grab my eye drops and moisten the eye about every hour. If I forgot to do that, my eye felt like it had glass shards in it.

CHAPTER 8
DEAR DIARY

Dear diary, Can I take this one more day?

I made it out of bed, I need to brush my teeth.
So I stumble and I reach out as I try to make it to
the sink.

I feel like I have had a thousand shots of whiskey,
but I haven't had a drop to drink. It's just my mind
trying to fix me.

It's like I'm standing on a boat and everything is
spinning. I'm swaying back and forth and the the
waves are unforgiving.

Can I take this one more day?

It's like everything is in motion, and everything is
loud. On the Inside it's ringing and the outside is
cranked for a crowd.

I can close my eyes and I can plug my ears,
but there is no escape from this misery or it's dry
tears.

I wish everyone would just shut up and I want the
world to stop moving. Sometimes this battle seems
like it's not worth winning.

Can I take this one more day?

I want to crawl under the table and I want to curl up and hide. I'm scared of the dark and the light blinds my eyes.

I look in the mirror, and I pull out loose hair, oh my God, my head is killing me. God, do you care?

My face is broken, and my nerves are in high def, I try to stay positive but I am scared to death.

Can I take this one more day?

My eyes are aching, just keep them closed. Imagine your life, the one your memory knows.

But, I can't even think, I can't concentrate. I feel paralysed and lost. Will this last forever? Is this fate?

Can I take this one more day?

I have lost so much weight and I can't taste my food. My taste buds are gone and I'm in a bad mood.

What is this reflection that used to be mine? Stapled, stitched, and lifeless, I'm not me, I'm a frankenstein.

Can I take this one more day?

Staring at my hands as I am on the shower seat, a bunch of loose hair lay at my feet.

Now I have a bald spot because my hair is falling out. I'm feeling less like a human and filling up with doubt.

Can I take this one more day?

I keep thinking I will wake up and it will be a happy day. But everything still sucks and I can barely find my way.

Everything repeats over and over. Madness and patterns are spinning out of order.

Can I take this one more day?

Nightmares never ending, nothing makes sense in my mind. But I'll just take a pill and go to sleep, It will all be just fine.

Everyday I think I can't go on, but here I on my bed I lay. I've survived this far, so maybe, just maybe, I can make it one more day.

I hear everything and nothing, my mind is lost, and food tastes like dirt. But I need to be strong and positive because healing takes a lot of work.

I CAN take this one more day.

CHAPTER 9
DOCTOR, HELP!

It wasn't long before my beloved sleep vacations were turning into nightmares. I was actually having more like night terrors. I would wake up in the middle of the night with my heart pounding and my body soaked in sweat. Now day or night, I was feeling tormented and overwhelmed. Thoughts of ending it all would run through my mind for a moment here and there.

At my follow up appointment, I had an MRI to recheck my brain. Everything looked good and I was to return in about a year for a recheck. I told my surgeon that I had started having more nightmares. My husband commented that he tried to wake me during the nights because I would be twitching in bed. I don't remember that, but I do know the dreams started coming and they were leaving me exhausted. And I went on to tell the surgeon I was exhausted, not sleeping, and basically miserable. That is when he diagnosed me with postoperative PTSD (Post Traumatic Stress Disorder). He explained that I might have outbursts of crying, anxiety, overstimulation, claustrophobia, fear of being alone, and of the dark. I pretty much had all those things.

He suggested that I try to let my mind work through it before trying any medication. He explained that although I was asleep for 12 hours, and I didn't literally remember having the surgery, my brain was very aware that it was being traumatized. It remembered everything. My subconscious mind was in turmoil and trying to find its way. My brain was panicking.

DAY BY DAY

I took the doctor's advice and tried to let my mind work itself out. I got plenty of rest, and would take quiet time just to meditate on things and let the feelings come out. I would cry and then feel better. I embraced the emotions, let myself feel them, and moved on. I tried to have a different view of myself. Instead of wallowing in my misery, I tried to be more grateful for the healing I was given and the family I had. I even went vegan because I even had a new view of animals. I seen them as lives, not food. Precious lives. In some odd way, I could relate to being trapped and prepped for slaughter. I suddenly understood many things differently.

I started walking more, doing yoga, and stretches. And guess what?! My facial nerves slowly started to come back. I had a crooked smile, but a smile all the same. And this gave me hope. I still had my bad days but I felt like the sun was rising.

Maybe I was going to be okay after all. My husband would take me by the arm and we went shopping. My husband pushed me even further and got me to try driving again. My balance was improving and my dizziness was subsiding. So we took little drives just down our little road. And it felt amazing. I felt like a human again. I started to get excited about life and was thankful I was still here and that I never gave up on myself. I got this burst of energy in my soul. In fact I was so excited, that I started going back to work. I was an administrative assistant and did computer reports, invoicing, and other miscellaneous paperwork. I figured I could handle that. The bills were piling up and I was getting antsy, so off to work I went. Twelve weeks after surgery I was back to the grind. And that lasted about twelve more weeks before I started backsliding. I was getting stressed at work, losing my balance again, getting agitated and depressed.

There was a few weeks that my husband hurt his back and I had to help him get better. I lost a lot of sleep and slid even further back in my progress. Soon I was getting irritated at everything. Noise, people, touch, light, you name it.

I went back to my Doctor and broke down in tears as I spoke with him. It was humiliating but inevitable. I was at the edge.

I was then diagnosed with neuro-fatigue and sensory processing disorder. He said that basically I went back to work too early, on a half of a battery, and was stressing myself out, and my brain's filter was taking in more than it could process. My batteries were drained. Too many noises, feelings, and movements were too much to bear.

My doctor took me out of work again to recover and rest. I was prescribed a day pill for depression and anxiety, and an evening pill to help me sleep and calm my nerves. The medicine was helping but two weeks turned into four and I started to feel like I was never going to be normal again. I just missed life. Symptoms were returning and even getting worse, and this time I felt like I couldn't pin it down. I was just drained to the point of not caring anymore. I was irritated and I felt like I was losing the battle, drained and going mad. I put myself in a healing deficit.

<u>THE GNAWING</u>

So I guess this PTSD and overstimulation disorder is what I would call a gnawing inside of me. It still lingers today. It's like a darkness and irritation crawling around inside of my body. I can't meditate it away, or wash it away, or run from it either way. It's just there, eating me from the inside out. It's in my head, and it's in my body.

I want to take a scrub pad and scrub myself from the inside. Erase the madness and powerwash the feelings away. It's almost too much to bare, and nobody can help me get rid of it. I think there is only one way out. The unspeakable thoughts run through my mind. I can't live like this anymore, but I can't leave my family in sorrow. I want to rip myself down to nothing. I want to pull my hair from my head, and I want to do it violently. The pain would probably be a relief just to distract me from the gnawing for a little while. Everything is overstimulating. Light, noise, and people. It is all gnawing me into fists. My nerves are vibrating with anger under my skin. I don't want to be touched, I don't want to be consoled, hugged, or loved. I just want to crawl under the table, plug my ears, and block the world out. I want a blank and black atmosphere with no movement or stimulation. I want stillness and peace.

But the gnawing stays. It is always there. It never relieves and it always wins. It's attached to me like a shadow that has crawled inside of my body and is running it's fingers along my nerves and veins. The gnawing climbs all the way up to my brain and says..."You died."

I died that day. My head was cut open, my mind silently fought for itself for over 12 hours, trying to grab hold of my body and shake it awake, but the anesthesia held it down with straps and tricks. My body was asleep, but my brain was screaming for help. And nobody could hear it. Not even me. I was oblivious, my person was being saved by doctors, while my brain remembered everything. And it remembered it like this... In the dark, cold room, I was sawed open, and parts of my head were removed, and parts of my head were replaced, and my mind subconsciously remembered it all. It was traumatized and it was trapped. My mind believed it was under attack. And it was defenseless. It was held down and it was violated.

I had to learn to retrain my mind. Calm the gnawing, and earn my own mind's trust. It seems surreal to say this, but it felt like I and my mind became two different people. And I had to heal this other person, who was a part of me. My mind had a mind of its own. Maybe that's what the subconscious is? I do not know, but it was all too mysterious, agonizing, and also amazing to feel like I was, in a way, seperate from my own self. On the outside I was me, and I had some control and some personality of myself, but secretly, inside, I was gnawing at myself. My mind could not cope with it's own memories. It was like a person chews on their nails when they are nervous, except my nerves were gnawing at themselves in madness. It felt like I had restless leg syndrome in my mind, and in my skin, and in every fiber and cell of my being.

It was unbearable, torturous, and maddening.

ALIVE OR ANIMATED
DEAR DIARY

Dear Diary, what have I become?

My body is moving but my mind is somewhere else. I'm in an unknown place. Uncharted territory in my mind. Almost as if everyday is a dream or even a memory, but my body is in a coma. I feel animated as if manipulated with strings and props. My face is paralyzed from surgery and I use my fingers to form a smile in the mirror. I try to brush my teeth but the water just runs down my face. My hair has thinned and is balding. Staples protrude down the left side of my head. My hands shake as I attempt to run my fingers across them. I sob... who is this girl I see? Where have I gone? I feel like the me that I once knew, that me, she floated away on that operating table, and what remains is this frankengirl.

I don't feel life inside me. I feel I have been taken away. And whatever has taken me is animating me. And while my body is animating through each day, my mind has terrible thoughts, dreams, and confusion. The world is spinning as my husband leads me through the halls to my bed. He tucks me in and my anxiety starts to take over as my brain thinks back to the cold place. The operating room. I don't remember it. But my brain remembers all too well. And so bedtime is a time for nightmares. Not nightmares of sad or scary stories, but unexplainable images that repeat over and over and over with no escape. I try to wake up but my body is disconnected. I just wait in torment for someone to shake me awake as visions of bloody veins and branches smother my mind. They crawl and grow around the inside of my head until they have completely covered any escape. They say that there is no waking up. And as my heart races and body twitches, my husband finally wakes me in concern. And I gasp in thankfulness to be woken from the dream's clutches. But then the room starts spinning again. My head is ringing, I can't hear or feel my head and face. So both day and night are torment over and over. Everyone is animating me through the day. Getting me dressed, helping me eat, helping me get to the bathroom. I can hear my heart beating loudly in my head. Bump, bum, bump...and ringing at the same time. My soul is a glass cage looking out at a spinning world. God help me. Because that big tree in the backyard and a long rope are starting to feel like a way home. And an end to this madness.

ACCEPTING THE MISERY

Two more weeks past and my medicine was helping me sleep enough to feel refreshed in the morning.

I would still be drained by about 3 pm, but somehow I kept myself going. And I think I came to a place of just accepting that this was my life now. I was going stir crazy sitting at home waiting for a magic ray of sunshine, so I insisted on going back to work. The doctor hesitated but agreed to every other day or half days. And I was to report any backsliding.

With the death grip on the steering wheel, I went back to work. I did my best to be mom, wife, and zombie. But truthfully, I was a carcass. I just made the motions of each day pass and I tried to flow with whatever the day brought. I'm fine... Yes, I took my pill..., yes, I slept..., no, I'm not over doing it... Blah, blah, blah... Bills had to be paid and I was sick of everything. My surgeons said this is to be expected, my MRI is fine, and so I just sucked it up and got into animation. It started to feel like it didn't matter how I felt or if I wore myself out to death, life just had to continue. Chores needed to be done, money had to be earned, and I was tired of complaining and feeling like a burden. So life spins, and my mind buzzes, I walk drunk, I get exhausted, and nobody really knows what is going on inside of me. For the sake of my family, I just submit to this new me. This animated and unforgiving life.

THE INVISIBLE SICKNESS

Today I realized that everything lingering inside of me, my irritation, my depression, the overstimulation, the aggravation... it's all invisible to the ones I love. On the outside I still look like LaWanda. I smile and act like LaWanda. But inside, there is this dark little corner where torment lives. And no one can see or feel it but me.

I have learned to cry in my mind, take deep breaths subtly, and mask pain and sadness with a tricking smile or joke. I have mastered pretending to be me. But I have a condition. And my condition is invisible. I can't explain it well, and I can't share it. My body went through it, my mind remembers it, and nobody can begin to know it or make it ok.

I take the pills, I see the doctor, and I talk to my husband, and it helps for a moment. But then the smallest thing triggers the dark corner back again and it never truly goes away.

My mind is different. I forget things, and most of it I don't even mention, because it is embarrassing. I run into things and hurt myself, and cover the bruises. Because everyone laughs and takes it like a grain of salt, but inside it scares me to death.

My skull tingles and my deaf ear buzzes. I can't hear half the things I need to, and I do hear the things that are miniscule.

My mind feels numb most days. Like I am in a daze. I sleep drive and don't remember how I got home half of the time. The days just pass. And I feel like a ghost walking right by the world around me. Sometimes I feel like I died and my soul is just hanging around like a lost shadow. Invisible. Sick. And just playing along. I'm not really here, and people don't really see me.

I haven't conquered this madness inside of me. But I am surviving it. I don't know how, and I don't know if it's forever, but I am here. Trying to enjoy the times that count, and make them worth more than my darkness. I have good days and I have bad days. I laugh , and I smile, but I'm not me. And when I am alone, I go to a dark place. I thank God that I am still alive. My surgery and recovery for the most part were a miracle. But I still feel broken.

Everyone's kind words are appreciated, and people try to help me through and see the bright side of things. But they don't see the inside. The place that is invisibly maddening. But each day brings its own hope and sometimes improvements. I hope anyone else who goes through anything similar to me, holds on tight.

And know that each day brings a new piece. And maybe someday this puzzle will be whole again, but until then, I make the best of what I can. And I try to have faith. I think back to the zebra, the black and white zebra. And the balance that I must keep in order to accept the new me and the dark place in my mind. That place in my brain that needs healing. That place I call... *The Pit*.

<u>CHAPTER 10</u>
THE PIT

There is no falling into the pit by accident.
One unknowingly and joyfully climbs down into it.

It starts in the tunnel, A colorful, bright, and happy tunnel. Full of promises, melodies, and memories. You are given a crayon and you are laughing and smiling. You take to the tunnel. Unknowingly and pitiful, you, like a nieve lamb, are lured unto its dreadful end as you joyfully and happily skip through the tunnel. You are not even fathoming what awaits at the end. You have your crayon and you run it along the wall as you skip and hum like an innocent child. There are many pictures of happy things colored along the tunnel.

After some time, the pictures begin to become scary and you are beginning to feel claustrophobic. Whispers enter your ears and slowly the tunnel becomes eerie, and the happiness has faded away.

Your skipping slows to a paranoid creeping toward a dark jagged edge. A tear runs from your eye and your chest tightens. Your heartbeat becomes a drum and it is unforgiving. You turn around and realized that the tunnel was just an illusion. Your mind has been tricking you. It gave you a moment of happiness. Enough to keep you sane for just a little longer. But the tunnel was just a bridge to the pit. It was easy to get into the pit. But turning around and leaving feels impossible. You have ran so far now. The only way through is to crawl down and get into the pit. You think to yourself that you might as well get into the pit and make the best of it. Then, you can go to the tunnel again. After all, maybe it was also an illusion? Or a test? Or is this all real? Was this really the pit or will your feet land on soft warm sand by a beautiful ocean?

But it is as you fear. A dark place made of cold and slimy brick. Musty waters and dead swamp creatures float about the pit. You stand in the pit shivering and clenching your eyes, only hoping to wake up. But you are alone and your thoughts are tormenting. You don't even try to crawl out of the pit. You know it has its hold on you. The worms crawl in and out between your toes. Why don't you leave the pit? Surely it is dark and cold. It holds no love, promise, or reason. But your mind played tricks on you and so you stay and pretend to be happy. You play in the mud and you name the creatures. You just sit and play in the devastation all day. You don't try to leave, You don't try to fight. Pleading does not scream from your lips.

 You count the bricks, You count the creatures, You inspect your skin, and anything else to stay occupied. There is no leaving and there is no sleeping. It is just you, cold, tired, and full of anxieties. You smile with tears and then cry laughing as you go mad. But finally, at that dying

moment, the waters begin to drain under your feet. The drums stop and you wipe your hair from your face. You look down at the floor, a grate of dead worms, vines, and sludge. You clench your eyes tightly and then open them to plainly see the bottom of your bathtub and all the smashed mushy crayons. The shower walls colored with pictures of happiness and scribbles of anger. Was the pit real?

"In the mind, everything is real. And only those who travel it experience its trauma."
-LaWanda Beyer

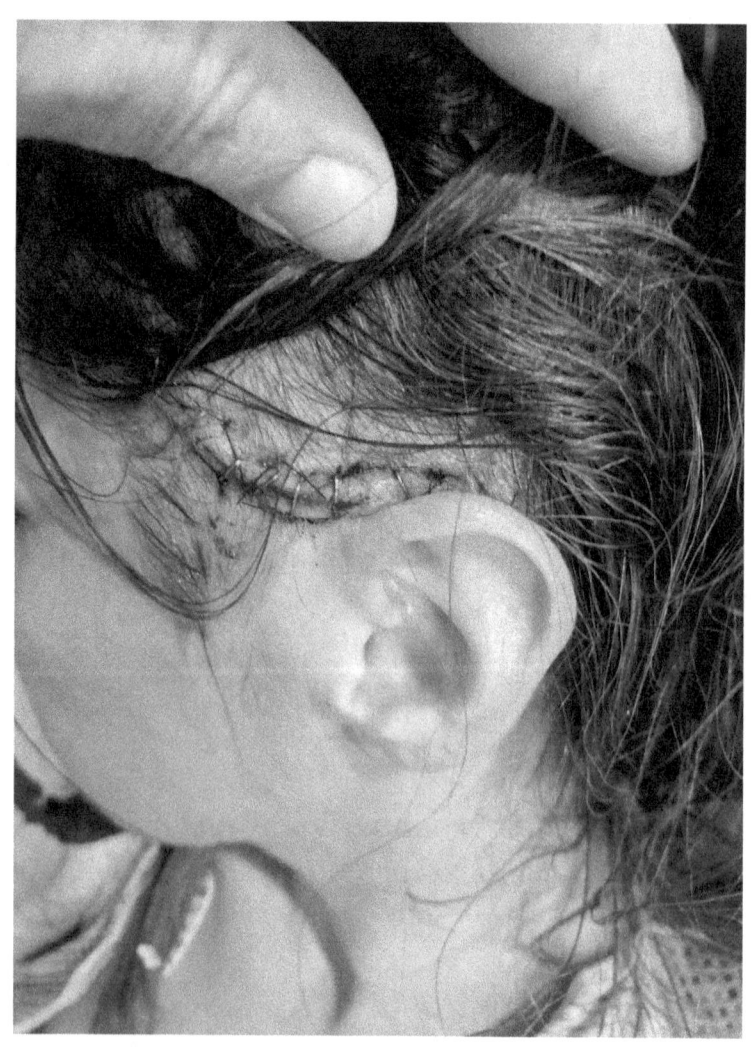

58

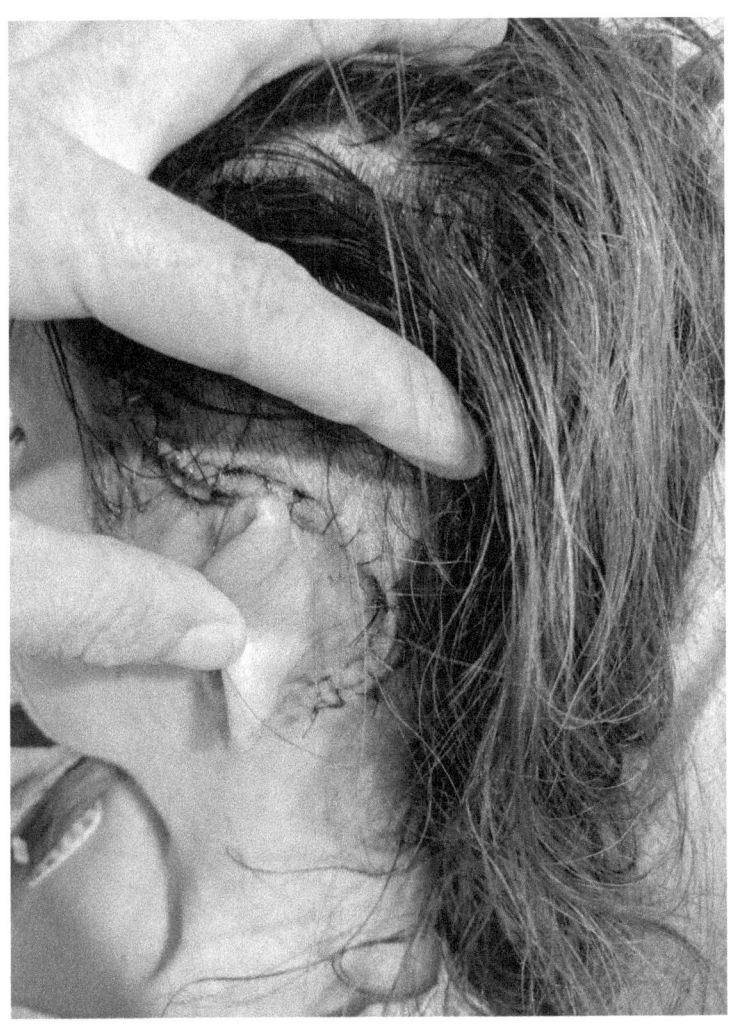

One day I will rise from this pit and escape this madness. I know it will take time and a lot of hard work, but by the grace of God, I will get there for I heal more everyday. It might be just a little, and it might be inch by inch, but I'm grateful, and I'm making it, and my God is with me.

I will rise from the madness. And that's a story for another day...

EXTENDED VERSION

ONE YEAR LATER...

At the time of writing this, It's been exactly one year now since I had my brain surgery.

It was obvious a year ago that I would have a difficult recooperation. The doctors said it would be tough. But it went far beyond what I ever had expected.

I can say today, that I was not prepared. I went out in a battlefield unarmed and naked. I wish I would have been more prepared and aware of what I was in for. Not that it would have changed the fact that I needed the surgery, but maybe I would have been a little more emotionally prepared.

Every day still brings some kind of emotional struggle. And some days it seems like there is no finish line from this madness. But, I drudge on with each passing day. Some days are good, others bad.

Sometimes I am so tired. It's like I have been treading water for days and I feel like I am jumping hurdles just to keep my heart pumping.

I find myself exhausted at the end of each day.

Sometimes just smiling and trying to be a "normal" person leaves me drained. And I feel outside of myself, looking in. And in my own way.

I don't want to cook or clean, or go out and do fun things. I actually feel my best when I am just sitting in my car. I don't know why. It is just a small space and a quiet place that I can just sit and be. Sometimes I just gaze into nothing, and sometimes just cry.

My husband will ask me, "What is wrong?"... and all I can say is, "I don't know. Everything. And nothing. But, just everything."

Do you ever just feel like you're screaming inside? You don't know why. You just feel trapped inside of yourself like you are in an emotional prison. No one can hear you and nobody has the key. You are just alone inside of your own mind. Waiting to die. I know that sounds awful, but the world is just rotating around you in slow motion. There is no such thing as time or priorities. There is just this paralyzing emotional blurr.

Sometimes I feel guilty, like I should be more grateful. But it isn't that I am not grateful, because I am. I am grateful to be alive. I am grateful for my physical healing. I am grateful to God, and I am grateful for my family. I am grateful just to be here. I know that I am lucky. My mind just feels like it never completely came home. It's stuck in a loop.

People ask me how I am doing. What do you want me to say? I am fine? I am doing good? Or even wonderful? What do I say in that awkward moment when someone asks me how I am doing? Nobody has the time to sit and hear what I really have to say, or what weighs heavy in my heart, and what torments my mind.

Nobody can fathom the emotional turmoil that struggles inside of me every day. Who really wants to hear it? Even if I took a month to explain it. If we sat and had 700 cups of coffee, their day would then go on, and mine would be unchanged. So, you see, it is just easier to say that I am doing good. And keep that box closed. I am never okay and I haven't the energy to explain it to you.

On a good note, physically, one year later, my facial nerves are still twitching. That's a good sign. It means that my body is still trying to heal. I am grateful for that. Most of my facial paralysis has healed. I have been so very fortunate to have survived the surgery and to have recovered physically as well as I have. And I am grateful, ever so grateful. I still get stabbing pains, shooting pains, and headaches. But oddly, wearing hats does help. Just a little pressure around my head brings some comfort.

My balance has greatly improved. I can drive and go to the store by myself. But if I get over tired, I start running into things and veering off when I walk. When I get like this, I don't drive. The best remedy for me is to sleep.

Sometimes I get short and quick moments when the room will spin just once. Then it's gone.

My tear ducts are still not working. The surgeon seems to note that it may be permanent. So I continue to put eye drops in multiple times each day.

 But emotionally, the battle still drags on. Maybe the emotional issues have hit me so hard because of the mental issues that run in my family? I have read this is a possibility. There is depression, anxiety, bipolar disorder, and even schizophrenia in my family history.

I know some people have this surgery and come out fine. Everybody's circumstances, reactions, and healing abilities are different.

I had other traumas in my life before I had this surgery. Maybe it all piled up and now I am just feeling the impact all at once?

Nineteen years ago I lost my baby girl. At five months of pregnancy, her lungs weren't developed enough to live. My water broke and by the time I got to the hospital her umbilical cord was hanging out of me. There was nothing they could do. I felt her kicking inside of me when the doctors told me I had to push her out. And by the time she came, she was gone. I will grieve her for a lifetime. That is just one of many traumas I had in my life before I even went through brain surgery. And I think that the trauma of losing her has resurfaced in my PTSD. And so now I have to deal with her loss or go mad.

I am going to include my book about *LOSING VICTORIA* in this extended version. As it is something I am now dealing with, along with other things that are surfacing from my brain. Things I tried to bury for years.

"How much agony? How much misery? How much trauma can one woman hold? With an amazing magnitude of emotional weight, I crawl through life. Bearing all, forgetting nothing, and feeling everything."

~ LaWanda M Beyer

Losing Victoria

A True Story About a Mother's Grief
And How She Copes

By LaWanda M Beyer

For permissions please contact author

www.lawandambeyer.com

Introduction

I lay on the floor gazing up at the swaying shadows on the ceiling.

The trees that stand outside the window dance as the breeze plays a peaceful melody.

I get lost in the motion and sound of the ceiling fan.

"Shwoosh...shwoosh...shwoosh..."

I close my eyes and drift into thought as I am taken back to the memory...

Soon the shwooshing starts to sound like a fetal heart monitor.

"Shwoosh. Shwoosh. Shwoosh."

A baby's heart beating from within the womb.

my chest fills with pressure as my heart begins to ache and Tears start running down my cheeks.

I keep my eyes closed.

I want to remember her.

I want to remember the sound of her heart beating.

I want to remember the feeling of her tiny feet
kicking inside of me.
Although the pain of losing her is too much to bear,
I have to feel it. I have to let the pain pass so I can
try to heal.

But it seems like the healing never comes.

I will always remember her, for she is a part of me.
Etched eternally into my soul.

The pain will never truly fade away and I don't
want it to. It reminds me that she existed.

It is the proof that I once held her...

even for a moment.

*"There is sympathy, sorrow, pity, empathy, and
compassion...
But, no consolation will bring comfort.
&
There is anger, despair, grief, misery, agony, and
anguish...
But, there is no name for the emotion that a mother
feels when she loses her child."*

Dedication:

The section of Losing Victoria, is dedicated to my beloved daughter,

Victoria Louise Beyer

&

My little brother,

Waylon James Anderson

May they be forever giggling in the arms of angels until we meet again.

Grief.

Everyone feels it. Everyone loses somebody they love. Everybody knows what it feels like to hurt inside because you miss someone dear.

I have lost people.

But the pain that a mother feels when she loses her child... it will sufficate you.

It is an unbearable emptiness.

Open hands with nothing to hold and
An empty womb with nothing to show.

Death pats you on the back as it rips the warm tenderness from your heart.

Turning back time

In the past I had many miscarriages. Mostly just a week or two along, but sad just the same.

I started to believe I would never have a baby.

One incident stands out in my head,
I was four months along, and I went in to have my check-up.

The nurse asked while smiling, if I had felt any kicking yet?

"No." I replied. And her smile faded away.

I didn't expect anything unusual as this was the farthest I had ever been along in a pregnancy.

She took her stethoscope and tried to listen for a heart beat. She moved it around many times.

I remember the anxiety that started to fill my heart.

Then she asked me to wait as they were going to do an ultrasound.

The ultrasound was then performed and i was not able to view the process.

I was then told to wait for the doctor.
 When he came in, one look at his face & I knew.

Something was wrong.

He said he was sorry but my baby stopped growing at nine weeks and it was not alive.

My body continued to believe everything was fine. My uterus was the size for being four months along and growing. Right on track. But the fetus was not.

Then, Ridiculously, I had to wait a week for an appointment to have a D&C to remove the fetus.

I had to live my life for a week knowing I was carrying my dead baby inside of me.

I was devastated.

I remember being curled up in my bed and holding my belly while I cried myself to sleep.

I prayed to god, and silently went insane.

But the appointment came and the appointment went, and time past.

I went through a phase where every month I was buying a pregnancy test.

I wanted a baby so badly.

It was the only thing that would fill this void.

I was grieving and obsessed.

finally

Finally the day did come when the test was positive again.

My doctor told me to take it easy. I had been through a lot.

Believe me, I was going to be the healthiest mama. I made sure I got rest, I ate healthy foods, and I prayed to God for my baby every night.

I stayed positive.

I talked to my belly, played it music, and believed that this time would be different.

It had to be. Or I would lose my mind.
Everything was going wonderful.
I was seven months along.

I had a big belly I was proud of, and I was so thankful for every kick, hiccup, and heartbeat.

One day, while visiting my mother-in-laws,

I was having contractions and lower back pain..

But it was early. Two months too early.

But we went to the hospital to be safe.

I was dilated to three. Instructed to take it easy. And go home. These things happen.

I took things easy, but a month later, we went in again with the same symptoms, just to be sure.

We arrived at the hospital. I was dilated to four & a half this time.

It was decided that This time we'll stay.

We walked the halls, and we will have this baby.

A month early, my son was born.

I had my son on november 24, 1997.

After many miscarriages, devastation, prayers, and hopes, he was welcomed into our life with open arms and great happiness.

I remember the day clearly, as most mothers do.

His beautiful face was a miracle.

His first cry a welcomed joy.

My heart was filled with emotions that did not exist.

Tears of pain and joy collided and I was forever transformed into a mother.

He had to be on oxygen for a day, otherwise was healthy as can be.

I made this tiny human and He was perfect.

Thank you god.
Seasons came and went.

It's one year later, and my little boy is my world.

 life was busy and I was ready to give grandma a burp rag and diaper.

I finally went back to work.

I Let my hair down, packed away the pregnancy clothes, and Joined humanity again.

 I was young. doing the fun things a girl can do when she is not pregnant.

I was waiting tables, and the love of my life was working two jobs. We struggled sometimes, but we were making it.

I had my man, my son, and life was good. Then...

<u>UtT-OhH</u>

One day, the signs of pregnancy crept upon me again.

Surely not again already? I thought.

as certain as the signs made themselves known, the test was positive.

Wow, did I ask for it or what?! And it wasn't that I wasn't grateful, but that void was filled, and I was not ready.

The past year I had learned that raising a baby is a big job. I was thankful and blessed, but...

this time I cried.

not in joy, but in selfishness.

I was not ready to have another baby.

I had just gotten myself back.

My body was finally back,
and so was my social life.

Shamefully, I was bummed..

My husband calmed me with his sweet words of
encouragement. He knew I was being absurd and
emotional.

"You can do this. This is good.
The kids would grow up together,
perfectly aged apart.
Why are you so down?"
He would ask.

I didn't know, I would say.

But that was a lie...

The hard cold truth... I didn't want to be home
pulling my hair out all the time, chasing two babies.
I wanted to be out with my friends more. I wasn't
ready to start all over again.

I was young, and All I was thinking about was
myself.

Time

Time changes things.

As I got deeper into my pregnancy, month by month, I became excited again. I got attached.

After all I had been through, how could I ignore all the reminders that a little life was growing inside of me. A little miracle.

Feeling those little kicks and hearing that tiny heartbeat.
I became grateful again.

Thank you God.

Why was I so hysterical before?

I felt badly for my initial feelings and selfishness as my baby moved about inside of me.

Then one day...

About five months along, my lower back was aching really bad. And I had pressure and aching in my girly area as well.

It felt like I was about to have a baby.

I called my doctor's office and they had me come in for an early check-up.

I drove an hour to the hospital and when I got into a room, I was told my doctor was gone that day. And the lady who seen me, a P.A., also obviously very pregnant, asked me about my symptoms. Then she told me to come back in a week to see my doctor, instead of my scheduled three week visit.

And no exam was performed.

I was angry that I drove all that way just to be told to come back in a week. But it must have been just normal?

Right?

But I was so uncomfortable.
I just didn't feel right.
But I went home thinking these must just be normal pregnancy things.

The aching continued.

Three days after my visit to the doctor, I was in the kitchen cooking and I sneezed.

When I sneezed, a gush of water came from me and it felt like something was coming out of me.

I ran to the toilet and wiped my legs and sat there while I called my husband to come get me. Quickly.

I told him, as I sat on the toilet, that I thought my water broke. And he insisted it was too early, and maybe it was just discharge...

"NO. no. NO! Get me to the nearest hospital because something is coming out of me!!"

I insisted angrily.

I felt like pushing but tried to ignore the urge. It felt like there was a ball inside of my canal, coming out.

I tried to urinate just a little bit and something fell into the toilet. I looked in fear as I stood up holding myself. There was no baby in the toilet. Thank God.

We hurried to the nearest ER where I was examined by the doctor on duty.

The doctor compassionately explained to me that my water had broke and what I had passed was my mucus plug.

I told him I was just at the doctor's office with complaints, but they did not check me.

He said that if this had been caught sooner, my cervix could have been stitched, and all would have been well.

But that was now not my case.

He said my baby's umbilical cord was hanging into my canal and there was nothing we could do but have the baby.

And he added that I should understand that at five months, my baby's lungs were not developed enough to survive.

That was just not acceptable.
My mind rejected the thought and my heart locked it's doors.

He asked if I wanted to stay at the hospital or be taken by ambulance to my regular doctor?

???.....HHmmm....??

In thinking that a second opinion would be good, I opted to be taken to my regular doctor.

I convinced myself all the way to the hospital that my doctor would save my baby.

I could feel her kicking inside of me.

When we arrived at the other hospital, I was carted to my own room. I was hooked up to monitors and tubes. I could hear my baby's heart beating and feel her kicking.

Unfortunately, Same story..
They said that she would not live.

But I did not believe them. I could hear her heart and feel her moving. She was strong and she was going to make it. I held my belly, feeling like this was all too familiar.

PUSH...

I pushed as my doctor instructed. And as I pushed I felt her kicking.

The nurse turned the heart monitor off.

I proclaimed that she was still kicking, she was alive!

Push again he said.

And with my last push, I felt one little kick and then she was out.

And the room was silent.

Time and existence stood still.

The doctor said he was sorry for my loss.

Everyone had somber faces as the nurse took my baby away.

I was in shock at this point. A barrier encapsulated my heart and mind. Walls went up. And I felt no emotion.

The world just rotated around me in slow motion as I was moved to a different room.

 I lay in the bed replaying the sound of my baby's heart beating over and over in my mind,
While the feeling of her kicking and moving haunted me.

Then a nurse walked into the room with a swaddled baby.

For a moment in time my heart leaped with joy.
They revived her!! I thought to myself.
Praise God!

But as she gently lowered my baby into my arms, and I saw her tiny body. Lifeless and cold.

I realized that this was not my hello.

It was my goodbye.

And I looked at her face.

 She looked just like her daddy.

Her tiny ears, nose, and fingers.

I looked at every detail.

Then, came the emotions.

Like a flood they drowned me and I was overwhelmed with grief.

I couldn't breath.

I was suffocating inside.

I asked the nurse to take her away.
I could not bear it another moment.
It wasn't real, but there she was lifeless in my arms.
I couldn't deny the pain. It was ripping me down to my bare begging soul, pleading to God for a miracle.

And then I lay there. With my empty womb and my empty arms. Warm tears on my cheeks, and an emptiness that I could not explain.

The hospital asked if we wanted a funeral.

I wanted one horribly, but we had no money, and the hospital said they could take care of her remains if we wished. And it would be done respectfully.

My husband just looked at me in my sad state and agreed for the hospital to take her.

I wanted nothing more than to just go home so I could curl up in a corner and die.

The hospital asked of her name.

Victoria Louise Beyer, I answered, with a quiver in my voice.

And they made her a crib card, bracelet, and took pictures of her to send home with me. None of which I wanted to even look at in that moment.

Going home

We left the hospital in silence.

We rode home in silence.

We left without a carseat.

We left without balloons.

We left without a baby.

We left a part of me behind.

In my mind, I screamed in silence...

Wait! Stop!

What if she is really alive?!

Wait! Stop!

I didn't hold her long enough!

Wait. Stop.

Go back...

Silently I screamed for her little body to be back in my arms. But the car kept on in silence.

Trees passed. Birds flew. The world kept turning, and we drove home.

Home was empty. There was an obvious missing piece. I looked around at everything that was still in its place when I left.

It Seemed like moments ago that I was just cooking right there and feeling her inside of me. And now she is gone. Just like that.

People apologized for the loss and went about their day.

I just thought to myself, how? How can the world even continue to turn without her in it?

Hating me

While feeling this emptiness, and reliving everything in my head, I remembered the beginning.

The day the test turned positive.
The day I was bummed.
Oh how I hated myself.

I never gave her the happy, warm, and welcoming feelings that a mom feels when she learns she's pregnant.

Her life was not celebrated in my heart on that day.

I was mad. I was selfish. I didn't want another baby.

On that day I found out I was pregnant, I cried.

Did she feel it?
Did she feel unwanted?

My mind was tormenting me. I am such a horrible person. I practically wished her away.
And now she is gone.

I want nothing more than to take that day back.

But I can't.

Is God punishing me?

Were my words and feelings on that day a curse that I placed on myself?

A lesson maybe?

Why didn't I hold her longer?
I should have held her for eternity.
I should have tried to talk to her.

But out of my own pain, I just handed her to a stranger.

How did I just leave her there?!
She wasn't a skunk on the side of the road. She was my baby!! And I left her little body there.

What did they do with her body?

Why didn't I find a way to give her a funeral? What kind of mother was I? Why didn't I speak up?

She deserved the most precious funeral...
She deserved roses from head to toe.
 She deserved words from a loving mother.

None of which she received.

I will live with regret and torment forever.

I think I was in such shock when I lost her, that I could not think of anything.

I couldn't make decisions, or answer questions.

My mother kept all of Victoria's things in her cedar chest. Having lost a baby herself, She knew I could not bear to look at them.

A tiny, green, poke-a-dot baby blanket that she was wrapped in, a crib card, a baby bracelet, and photos of her tiny and fragile body from head to tiny toes. All wrapped up in a bag.

And it was so...
I could not bring myself to even think about looking at her things without bursting into tears.

I didn't know if I ever could or would.

And I started to feel my heart turn cold, and angry.

Did I even ever deserve her.

Mad at the world

I had a few miscarriages before Victoria.
The loss of tiny fetus' at a few weeks along. And I believe that a baby is a baby as soon as that test turns positive. And I grieved for those babies.

But losing a baby that you actually felt moving inside of you, growing, and kicking for five months, was a different grief. A great loss of attachment.

I was bonded to this little life inside of me. It was as if I already knew her.

And so this time, when People would say that they were sorry to hear about my miscarriage...

I was angry.

Miscarriage?...

I didn't have a miscarriage.

I had a baby.

Her name is Victoria.

She lived, kicked, and had a name.

She was born, held, and died.
I held her in my arms and felt her lifeless body as it
kill me emotionally.

And why is nobody hurting as much as I am?!!

Why didn't that lady, the P.A., check my cervix
when I went to that appointment three days
earlier?!

If she would have just checked me, Victoria would
be here today.

Does she even know? or feel bad?
It was routine, why didn't she check me?!

Why didn't I demand a check?!

I miss her. And I am angry. I hate everyone. I hate myself.

Every baby I would see, every pregnant belly, every baby section at the store, and every December....

Brought the memories flooding.

Aftermath

Everytime I went to the doctor for a check-up, I was still bleeding.

The doctor said that it should ease up anyday.

He also informed me that I had an incompetent cervix. That basically my cervix was not strong enough to hold in a baby to full term. And if I ever became pregnant again, be sure to tell my doctor, as I would need a cervical cerclage. My cervix would need to be stitched shut.

This all came clear as I thought back at how I was dilated early with my son. And suddenly I felt thankful he even made it into my arms.

Each following appointment was the same...

Still bleeding.

Twelve weeks post delivery and I was still bleeding.

Just another reminder that I had a stillborn.

Finally the doctor said that all my bleeding was not right and he did a check of my cervix.

He said that there was a piece of placenta still attached inside. And he was going to remove it.

 As I lay there just waiting for him to finish, he called the nurse and informed her to prep for emergency.

He told me to just lay still and stay calm.

I didn't know what was going on.

The nurse rolled in a wheelchair. They told me to sit up slowly, not to be alarmed, but to get into the wheelchair.

I felt light headed.

They had to take me to the ER for an emergency D & C. (A scraping of my insides).

As I slowly sat up, the sight before me was devastating. There was blood everywhere, and I mean everywhere. His office looked like a slaughterhouse. There was An astronomical amount of blood on the exam table, his equipment, and his carpeted office floor.

I gasped, as my heart started racing with anxiety.

"Come on now", he said to me, while easing me into the wheelchair, "You are hemorrhaging quickly."

I heard him direct the nurse to rush me to the ER as swiftly as possible.

My mother was called in and I was rolled downstairs to the ER.

Along the way, the nurse kept looking under the chair to make sure we weren't leaving a trail. My wheelchair was covered in many pads and blankets.

My mother and the nurse kept nudging me. "Stay awake" they said.

I was starting to fall asleep. I felt weaker and weaker, nodding in and out with their poking and prodding.

The ride to the ER seemed to take forever. Like it was in slow motion.

Yet I hadn't a care in the world.

I felt peaceful, as if death was upon me.

I remember thinking... Go ahead, take me.
I deserve it. Take me from this world.

I wished my daughter away, so just take me.

I wanted to sleep and wake up with her in my arms.

I barely remember being in the ER. It all happened
so quickly. I remember the doctor coming in and
doing the D & C. I faded in and out of consciousness.

I remember him telling the nurse that there was no
time for pain medicine.

I layed there afterwards for a moment. In pain.

Then, suddenly, they said I could go home. I
remember thinking that it was some kind of joke.

But no, they stood me up on my weak legs. I could
barely stand, let alone walk.

They propped me up against the wall in the hallway
where I could barely stand or focus mentally.
I felt as if I was going to just pass out.

My mother came rushing to assist me. I remember
her anger.

She was in disbelief that they just threw me in the hall like a lame animal ready to die.

Like they were trying to get rid of me as soon as possible.

I had lost so much blood, was so tired, and unhappy that they didn't just let me die.

I must have told my mother that,
because I remember her saying that it was just the blood loss talking.

I looked up and my husband had finally gotten to the hospital. I remember him walking towards me. He was confused with what was going on. All he knew was that I had a check-up that day.Then he received a call from the doctor's office saying I was in the E.R.

He took me home,
where I went to bed and slept for a long time.

I was wiped out.
Exhausted and depleted.
Physically & emotionally.

My mother was very upset, insisting that I should have had a blood transfusion.

That was the last time I ever dealt with that hospital. And I never seen that doctor again.

Some thought I should have sued for not getting my cervix checked when I complained of my pain and symptoms. If they would have done their job, and seen that I was dilating, Victoria would be here today.

And maybe I should have. But it didn't matter to me. No amount of money would bring her back to me. Or bring me any relief or replacement.
The damage was done.

<u>Carrying on</u>

The bleeding gradually slowed and came to a stop. Finally.

Life for me was not the same after losing Victoria.

There was always an emptiness.

Although another baby would never take her place, I started yearning for another baby.

I wanted the feeling back.
I wanted to hear a heart beating, and I wanted to love a baby as soon as the test was positive.
I wanted to hold it, love it, rock it, and appreciate it.

But it was the grief. The trauma, and the pain talking to me.

I had my son and I was grateful for him even more than ever.

But still.. The anguish of losing Victoria would not leave.
It wouldn't even be merciful.

I carried the pain and loss in my heart silently.
Every day.

Thinking no one would understand,
I would cry alone in my room.
Then I would hold it in and carry on.
There was no healing.

I would get mad at God, mad at my husband, mad at everything. I just wanted to punch something. I was festering.

Twenty years Later

Twenty years later, I still have my son and another Daughter. I was blessed with another baby girl years after Victoria. And she is and always will be, my sunshine.

But nothing replaces Victoria.

Twenty years later, Victoria's things are still in that bag and I can't bring myself to look through them.

The mentioning of her name brings me to gasping tears to this day.

And every December, on the anniversary of her birth, I silently mourn for her alone.
Just days before Christmas, my child was not born.
Christmas changed.

HEALING

On August 18, 2017, I went through a surgery to remove a brain tumor. The devastation of it left me with postoperative PTSD.

My brain was traumatized.

I have recovered physically from the surgery, but emotionally, I am still suffering to this day.

Things from the past have come to the surface as my brain tries relentlessly to heal.

And I realized while trying to recuperate,

that I have so much trauma carried within myself.
And I really needed some emotional healing.

Emotional baggage was wearing me out to the
point of thinking about killing myself.

And losing Victoria was damage within me that
took up half my secret pain baggage.

A bag full of emotional pain that I swung over my
shoulder everyday. And it was weighing me down
with regret, grief, anger, and blame.

I decided I need to get this out and recover.

I needed to heal.

I realized that healing wasn't forgetting. I didn't
have to forget her, I just needed to release the pain
of her.

I needed to be able to say her name out loud
without breaking down in tears. I needed to stop
blaming myself. Stop mourning her memory,
and start celebrating that I had her. If for even a
moment.

I needed to bring positivity to her memory. Cherish
her name.

My first step in attempting to heal was to acknowledge that she was ever here, and talk about her out loud. To people, or to just myself. I needed to talk about her or to her while folding laundry or washing dishes. I just need to say her name and tell my brain that it was okay to uncover her memory.

I sat one day and told my daughter about her. Of course I cried and my heart felt like it was going to explode, but it felt good afterwards to have spoken her name. It felt like I breathed life into her memory.

I needed to do this more. No more burying pain. No more suffering in silence.

I decided to do affirmations.

Standing in the mirror, I told myself out loud, speaking to my reflection:

~I forgive myself
~I forgive the P.A. for not checking me.
~I forgive God.
~It wasn't my fault.
~I'm not being punished.
~I will heal.
~She is giggling with the angels.
~I will see her again someday.

~She knows that I love her.
~She knows that she was wanted.

I found that keeping a diary and writing about my feelings helped tremendously. Especially on days when I didn't feel like talking, but had a lot on my mind.

Just writing this book and getting this all off my chest has made a big impact in my healing.

Then, one day, while writing, I thought to myself... Why not write a letter to Victoria?

It took me a long blank stare into my screen before I could start a letter to my beloved baby, but I did it.

And afterwards, I felt a sense of relief and comfort. I felt as if she heard me.

I will share my letter with you...

Dear Victoria,

My precious baby, know that I never meant for you to be taken from me.
Even though I was not ready for another baby so soon, I would have never, ever, chosen to give you up, send you away, or wish you gone.
You were wanted with all of my heart and being. If you were here today, I would never let you go. I would hold your little hand forever.
You are embedded into my heart and I hope that you can feel my love for you.
I am sorry that you were taken too soon.

We never got to grow together, laugh together, or experience anything together, except separation.
I hope and pray that you did not suffer when you left this world.
It kills me not knowing if you know how much I love you. So, know that I love you with all my heart and all my soul.
You are my precious angel.
You are my baby.
I will love and miss you until the end of my days.
I believe that one day we will meet again.
And on that day, I look forward to holding you in my arms.

Until then, and with all my love,

Mom

Although all my tactics for healing didn't help completely, I did find some relief.
 But I still mourn her.

I think there is relief to be found in these practices, and healing does improve more with time, but a mother's grief doesn't ever truly go away.

It's 20 years later, and I keep looking at that box that holds the bag of Victoria's things. And I am getting up the nerve to visit it one of these days. And I know that when I do, as soon as I open that bag and start pulling things out, it is going to be like it happened yesterday.

And so I procrastinate.

One year later, I battle with my demons, and I am working on accepting the new me.
I'm getting used to being half deaf, having pains, and dry eyes. My doctor says that my PTSD may never completely go away. I avoid loud places that overwhelm my mind. Overstimulation has improved, but is still here. But this is the new me, and i am grateful I have some progress, can function, and be here for my family.

Author's Note

Friend & Reader,

If you have lost a baby or child in any way, or gone
through a trauma that is beating you down,
I feel your anguish.

Let's keep our chins up as we push through this
trauma together.

Try some exercises to ease your discomfort.
Talk to your family, doctor, and/or a therapist.

Don't stand silent in your pain.
Don't hold in your grief alone.
It only festers & makes the pain worse.
Try to Find your place of peace
and celebrate life when you can.

Healing is not forgetting, healing is accepting..

*"A baby is a treasure unmeasurable
and a loss inconceivable.*

*I can still feel her tiny, dainty, and fragile body in my
arms.*

Losing her will always be my emotional prison.

And I will grieve her for a lifetime."

~LaWanda M Beyer

MY GREATEST THERAPY

Amazingly, my greatest therapy has been writing this book. I kept notes and diaries along the way and they ended up becoming the book you are reading right now. And I have continued to write.

Growing up and to this day, I hated reading. You wouldn't catch me with a book EVER. But writing, well that is a different story. Since writing this book I have found a secret passion. I never would have thought I would like to write so much, but now it's all I think about. It brings me relief and takes me outside of my head. So I guess in a way, this pain and experience has brought out a new me, and a new passion.

Everytime I write, I feel a door open inside of me and it's like the room gets all swept out. My anger, sadness, frustration, and stuck emotions can come out in a story. I open my imagination and expel my feelings into pages. It doesn't have to be my story. It doesn't even have to be real, it just needs to escape. And so I have found this outlet. This emotional loophole, in my writing. So I encourage others to find their loophole. Maybe it's not writing, or maybe it is. Maybe it's in music, painting, crafting, or volunteering. But find it.

Rise above the madness.

If you can't find your you again, then maybe it's time to be new.

Don't get me wrong, I am not magically some healed girl with a talking grasshopper in my pocket. Rainbows are not falling on my head and my footprints are not leaving glitter behind. But, I am a little better emotionally, since I started writing.

And even a little bit is a lot when you feel like nothing.

ABOUT THE AUTHOR

Hello. My name is LaWanda. I am a wife, mother, pet lover, and author. I am a haphazard girl. A lover of folklore, adventure, imagination, and life.

In 2017 I underwent the deepest cranial surgery that a person could have. I had a tumor removed that was pressing on my brain stem. The recovery from the surgery along with its symptoms nearly drove me mad. During my recovery process I started keeping notes and diaries of what I was going through. Then, I decided to publish it all as a book for others to understand what a loved one might experience. Writing the book was not just a way of getting my experience out, but it was also my therapy. It was an emotional ejection of bad thoughts and feelings.

In saying all that, my first book, *Reduced To Madness*, was born. It made top 100 best sellers in neurosurgery in its first month.

After my first book was published, I found that writing just flowed from my soul. I enjoyed it so much that I decided to keep going. I never knew I had this secret love of writing inside of me and how much relief it could bring to me in my healing. Going through the pain and madness of losing babies, brain surgery, and other traumas, in a way, has made me who I am today. A new person. A girl who just wants to drink her coffee with a warm blanket and release all her feelings and imagination from her mind into books.

I hope you enjoy or find comfort in some of my works. I have so many stories in the stirring pot, so please stay in touch, follow me on social media, and feel free to contact me.

www.LaWandaMBeyer.com

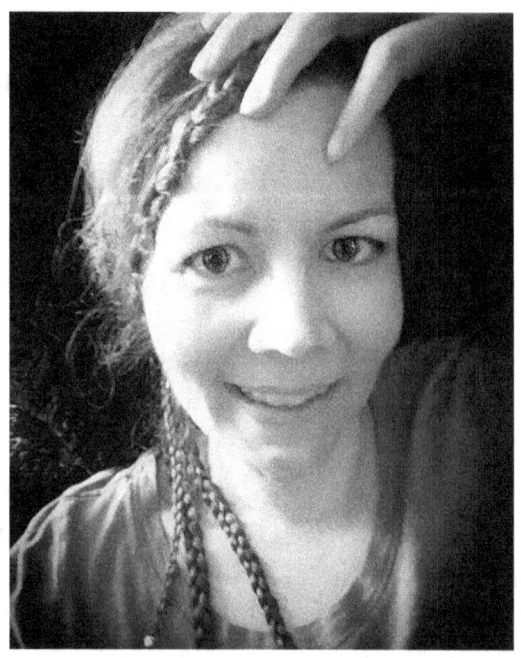